The Essential Clinical Social Work Series provides state-of-the-art theoretical and clinical knowledge for clinical social workers and other mental health practitioners.

Essential Clinical Social Work Series

Series Editor
Carol Tosone, School of Social Work, New York University, New York, NY, USA

Meredith Hemphill • Abigail Nathanson
Editors

The Practice of Clinical Social Work in Healthcare

Springer

Editors
Meredith Hemphill
City Center Psychotherapy
New York, NY, USA

Abigail Nathanson
Silver School of Social Work
New York University
New York, NY, USA

ISSN 2520-162X ISSN 2520-1611 (electronic)
Essential Clinical Social Work Series
ISBN 978-3-031-31649-4 ISBN 978-3-031-31650-0 (eBook)
https://doi.org/10.1007/978-3-031-31650-0

This Springer imprint is published by the registered company Springer Nature Switzerland AG
The registered company address is: Gewerbestrasse 11, 6330 Cham, Switzerland

Foreword

The theme of 2022's NASW celebration of Social Work Month is "The Time is Right for Social Work." The same can be said of this book. The time is right for a book that focuses on the educational needs of new and early social work practitioners in health care – one might say it's overdue. It can become a go-to guide for all of us when we begin our work with a newly diagnosed patient and their family.

This book is published amidst the COVID-19 pandemic, which has lent a sense of urgency to the work we do in health care. It was social workers, along with our nursing, physician, and chaplain colleagues, who rose to the occasion of providing bio-psycho-social-spiritual care to the legions of patients and families who dealt with the trauma of a little-understood disease that descended upon the healthcare system and on them without warning. The crisis of the pandemic highlighted the unique clinical nature of our work – the way we hold space for the myriad of feelings that arise when people are thrust into the world of illness. We often enter Arthur Frank's "chaos" narrative with patients and families – a story that cannot be put into words. Yet social workers in health care are often called upon to do just that: to help patients and families put their suffering into words, so that their stories can be understood and they can find a recognizable self. This book will help us in that journey.

The book's dual emphasis on chronic illness across the lifespan and the importance of a trauma-informed lens has much to teach us about coping with that chaos. The book is divided into disease-specific chapters, providing a guide through the unique challenges each presents. Using Rolland's psychosocial typology of illness, each chapter addresses onset, course, possible outcomes, and the degree to which the patient's functioning is affected. It also reminds us that the patient is part of a family system – family in the broad sense of the word – and that family members need care as well. It shifts the focus from symptoms to whole-person care. This framework can also begin to bring order to the chaos and give the new clinician practical information and a starting point.

All illnesses bring with them a sense of unreality and confusion. What has happened? How do I make sense of this new world I have entered? How can I feel safe in a body that has let me down? Trauma-informed care is not only for those that have come into our health system with a history of trauma. It is also a helpful framework for coping with all the small attacks on our sense of safety that even the best of healthcare systems inflict. For those who have suffered trauma prior to the illness, and/or have been marginalized and oppressed, trauma-informed care is an imperative. Social work, with its abiding commitment to social justice and to the dignity and worth of every individual, is *the* healthcare profession charged with centering these experiences and giving them voice.

Healthcare social work has been my abiding passion for 40-plus years. As a clinician, I have worked with thousands of patients and families who are facing serious, chronic, life-threatening, and terminal illness. As an educator, I have worked with an equal number of students and social workers who want to make a difference. It is heartening to me that many of them, beginning with the editors of this book and a good number of the book's authors, have been trained through New York University's Zelda Foster Studies Program in Palliative and End-of-Life Care. It is a fitting legacy to the memory of Zelda Foster, an early pioneer for hospice and palliative care, and a woman who always championed new ways of knowing and caring for patients and families.

Susan Gerbino
Clinical Professor and Director
of the Zelda Foster Studies Program
in Palliative and End-of-Life Care
New York University
New York, NY, USA

Preface

What does social work have to offer patients with serious diseases, illnesses, and conditions? Healthcare institutions are increasingly recognizing that *good care* isn't only about *good medicine* and *physical remedy*. It also involves caring for a person's mental, emotional, and spiritual welfare as they face physical challenges. It acknowledges that people exist outside of their diseases, and the diseases are not just happening to some cells in the body; they are happening to the entire person. As our entire selves are impacted by serious illness, so do our entire selves need to be the focus of care if proper care is to be provided. Healthcare social work, then, has a central role in the wellbeing of patients who are seriously and/or chronically ill. This book shares what we and our colleagues know about the interweaving of psychosocial and non-medical aspects of a patient's experience with serious illness.

The idea behind this book came from an earlier project in 2019, a special issue of the *Clinical Social Work Journal* that asked social workers in healthcare: *What does clinical social work look like here?* It was then and continues to be our opinion that *clinical* social work in healthcare is under-discussed in social work and medical literature. Lacking practical opportunities to use clinical skills learned in school in many parts of healthcare may leave social workers struggling with how to fine-tune their clinical expertise in a fast-moving, physical illness-focused environment.

What is meant by *clinical* social work in this book? *Clinical* pertains to the points of distress and psychosocial issues that arise in dialogue with physical illness, in addition to and beyond concrete service referrals. Clinical social work interventions tend to focus on the intra- and interpersonal dynamics of a patient and those around them; the meaning made of illness, survivorship, and death; and the shifts in identity and connection that often come with serious illness. These issues tend to appear alongside critical points in an illness journey (i.e., diagnosis, initiation of treatment, waiting, recovery, remission or recurrence, progression of disease, survivorship, or ongoing care). They are also determined by other health and psychosocial factors, such as: suddenness of onset; history of illness and/or familiarity/associations with the illness; co-occurring health or mental health issues; substance misuse; trauma history; and other life struggles. They can substantially worsen a person's experience of being ill and receiving treatment, and the experience of caregiving or bearing witness to the illness of a loved one.

While Maslow's hierarchy of needs supports the effort to secure physiological wellbeing and safety first, it does not suggest that wellness and wholeness happen at this level alone; basic physical survival is the bedrock to the rest of the human experience but not the only definition of it. Practical assistance is sometimes (erroneously) seen as our primary value in healthcare. In fact, our Code of Ethics calls us to attend to both practical and psychosocial issues when it reminds us of our responsibility to support and uphold the dignity and worth of our clients.

To imagine the import and impact of the *clinical* aspects of illness and care to a patient, consider this example:

> Melissa, a 35-year-old Latinx cisgender woman with an early-stage gynecological cancer, appears in high distress at every medical appointment. Her medical team is perplexed. They wonder aloud: *She has been told that she has a high probability of remission and cure following surgery and radiation. Why isn't she more positive? She has a great prognosis!* They refer her to their social worker for psychosocial assessment and assistance. Understanding that the patient's thoughts and feelings surrounding medical appointments cannot be assumed, the social worker explores them with Melissa. The social worker learns that she is very afraid and vigilant because she associates gynecological medical examinations with past experiences of sexual abuse. The social worker also learns that the patient dreads the medical interventions planned, fearing that they will bring back trauma memories or even retraumatize her. She admits that even though she knows it is probably not true, she sees the cancer as proof of her damage from the abuse. Far from looking forward to being cancer-free, the patient looked back and feared a return to the fragile psychological and emotional state that she experienced early on after her abuse ended.[1]

This is a striking example of how a person may face psychological barriers to care and feel harmed over the course of care, no matter how adeptly the medical care is provided.

The articles produced from *The Clinical Social Work Journal* special issue helped clarify our effort to define more fully the goal of "helping patients cope with illness." Having supported patients in various healthcare settings ourselves over a combined 30 years (several centuries when we aggregate the wisdom and experience of our authors), we know that this phrase can mean a lot, or very little. Coping with illness means more than coping with the reality of a physical limitation or symptom. Looking more deeply, we can understand it to mean: How do we cope with waiting and uncertainty? How do we cope with inadequate disease-modifying treatments and prognostication? How do we stay a recognizable version of ourselves throughout our illnesses? How do we reckon with old, unresolved issues that have re-emerged, triggered by illness? How do we recognize our positionality within the social and political constructs that define treatment and healthcare, and react to and cope with the navigation of disease/symptom treatment within those constructions?

---

[1] All names and other personal identifiers in this case are fictitious. Any similarity to actual persons, living or dead, or actual events is purely coincidental.

How healthcare social workers define a person's *struggle to cope* depends on what they see their specific patient population face most often. Social workers may expect patients who had heart attacks to experience coping difficulties related to the suddenness of onset, whereas patients with diabetes may be expected to struggle to cope with the slow and ongoing nature of monitoring and care. Likewise, the interventions and approaches social workers take in healthcare can vary, in part because of different faces of illnesses and corresponding definitions of *coping with illness*. It can vary depending on a social worker's position within their institution and the culture of their teams as it relates to the roles and expertise of social workers. It can also vary depending on the social work training and education received in preparation to support patients. Some social workers come to their first hospital position with field experience in such settings and masters-level education focused on related topics, like working with older adults, grief, loss, and bereavement. Others have less experience and education that can serve as foundations for patient assessment and work.

In this regard, healthcare social workers are distinct from many of the professionals with whom they work. While physicians and nurses tend to have highly structured, intensely role-specific training in their schools, social workers may find their training varies broadly. In our experience, it is common for social workers new to healthcare or new to a specific population feel a bit daunted and underprepared to deal with the full complexity of the psychosocial issues before them. A lot of learning happens "on the job," and is thus dependent on the ability and bandwidth of specific departments, supervisors, and teams to provide adequate clinical training to social workers beyond the mechanics of doing their jobs. In recent years, there are more opportunities for emerging social workers to deepen their clinical healthcare practice outside of psychotherapy training and to integrate the two themselves, and our hope is that this book will be part of that movement.

Patients may be referred to them with a specific disease, or several comorbid diseases. A social worker in oncology may feel very comfortable with their clinical skills in dealing with cancer, but benefit from a deeper understanding of how an event like a heart attack or diagnosis of dementia may look along similar psychosocial structures when their patients present with those issues as well. Equally, a social worker may find themselves assigned to a new specific population and benefit from an organized approach to better utilizing their existing skill set with a new group. A new social worker, meanwhile, may not know where to begin looking for direction on how to help.

We organized this book to add depth and uniformity to the topic of clinical social work practice in healthcare through the use of a clinically focused conceptual frame throughout. In discussion with Rolland's (1987) framework of illness and aging, we developed a frame that focuses on pertinent clinical issues, patient experiences, and emerging trends in medical social work across illness categories. Rolland's theory posits that the trajectory of an illness drives the family's experience of it, from a developmental, psychosocial lens. The nature of onset, for instance, whether acute (heart attack) or insidious (dementia), impacts how the patient and family cope and integrate the illness into their narratives. Consistent with this outlook, we examine how the phase of the disease intersects with the individual and familial development of the patient.

Each chapter is organized by illness, illness classification (diagnosis/onset, course, outcome, and degree of incapacitation), and then by common clinical issues seen in crisis, during treatment, during advanced disease, and at end-of-life and bereavement. We attempted to cover a range of illnesses that are medically and psychosocially impactful. We appreciate, however, that our list is incomplete. Chapters often combine diagnoses; when this occurs, it is because these health conditions/illnesses are considered to not necessarily have similar medical compositions and classifications but similar psychosocial stressors and patterns. Heart attack and stroke are placed together, for instance, because psychosocially they are associated with similar impacts and experiences, as do for heart and lung diseases, or kidney and liver diseases.

Applying systems theory (which understands that a person's life and personhood are negotiated in interaction with various relational, societal, and institutional systems), we include a social justice discussion in each disease chapter. The social justice sections examine how individuals belonging to particular demographic groups are potentially affected inequitably as they interact with systems of care, rules, and policies on their journey through their illness. The authors' reflections on clinical practice in each area add insights on clinical work with each patient group, insights that authors have arrived at in the field and through their research and writing on each group's hallmark psychosocial stressors.

Tables are included in many of the chapters to summarize the defining psychosocial characteristics of each illness or condition (see Table example). These tables are segmented by stages of illness, and accompanied by recommended areas of focus for clinical work (i.e., clinical goals and interventions). In some chapters, this same content is covered in the paragraphs rather than in table form; the example below may be a framework by which readers may understand the material throughout.

Table example Psychosocial issues and clinical goals and interventions

Phase	Psychosocial issues	Clinical goals and interventions
Crisis/acute	Long journey to diagnosis/unclear diagnosis Uncertain treatment course Initial impact of illness and prognosis	Coping with waiting, uncertainty, and fear Patient advocacy/follow through to establish diagnosis and treatment plan
Chronic	Long-term medical monitoring and treatment Related psychosocial changes Pain management Restricted quality of life Unpredicted/occasional symptom flairs	Psychosocial and emotional support for coping with range of possible health effects Validation of patient's mental health challenges and emotional experiences related to autoimmune disease
Terminal	If occurs, likely to induce despair and anticipatory grief Increase dependence on caregivers and other services, i.e., palliative care	Intensive support for physical symptoms Ease distress with strong support symptom for new mental and physical distress

With few exceptions, chapters are co-written by social workers at different points in their careers. Most paired authors come from different institutions and often did not know each other before this project; our intention was to encourage conversations about the assumptions and cultural values we each have. Our authors come from all across the country, and vary in race, age, ethnicity, gender identity, immigration status, and socioeconomic background, though all are at least licensed, masters-level social workers. COVID-19 has changed our experience of this book, and new research about the best provision of care comes out every day. We have strived to be patient-focused and trauma-informed, and to demonstrate cultural humility, yet we know there will be shortcomings, indicative of a process of learning and attunement that is never complete.

A note on the scope of the book and word choices throughout it. While we appreciate the import of the intersection of pre-existing mental health and substance use issues on serious physical illness, it is beyond the scope of this book to address the multitudinal psychosocial impacts that may arise as a result. We hope that future work focused on the possible psychosocial impacts of serious health issues for individuals with mood and personality disorders and substance use disorders will be written, as we see this, too, as an area needing further exploration for healthcare social workers today. We have also chosen to limit our scope on the age and developmental groups we discuss. In this book, we focus on the experiences of adults with illnesses, and children impacted by those adults' illnesses and treatment. As with mental health issues, we see the value of a contribution focused on the group we do not address – in this case, children coping with physical illness – and we hope to see more on this topic, using a clinically focused frame. And, concerning word choice: we have been diligent in our consideration of terminology and phrasing for this book. We refer to people with illness as "patients" intentionally, not to reinforce a paternalistic hierarchy but to acknowledge that this relationship is between a person who is physically ill and a provider of care, and is defined within the realm of healthcare provision. We limit the connotation that a person is heavily defined by their disease (X) or illness (Y) by identifying them as a person or patient with X or Y. Secondly, we use the term "caregiver" to mean any person impacted by the care of a person with a serious illness, whether the care is logistical (hands-on care or organizing formal care) or emotional (offering companionship or support as a family member or friend). Finally, we use the term "family" to mean either families of origin or families of choice and creation, with equal weight, depending on the circumstance of the person with serious illness. Along those lines, we use the term "family and friends" where other literature may refer to "loved ones," honoring the complexities of the relationships in which we provide care. With other phrases and terminology, we, as editors, have often chosen to honor the expertise and perspective of the authors.

An important feature of this book is an approach on trauma-informed care in healthcare. While most people have at least a cursory understanding of the discrete "big T" traumas (war, assault, accidents, etc.), as they are colloquially referred to, the impacts of developmental, interpersonal, and other "little t" traumas (interpersonal conflict, relationship loss, childhood neglect, etc.) are often less discussed and understood. Further, the overlap of how we understand trauma in terms of coping with a threat to the self has significant overlap with how we understand illness as the same; in healthcare social work, the questions then arise: How do we encourage people to stay present in their bodies when their bodies are the site of the threat and discomfort due to illness? How do we ask people to give or receive care, when that requires a vulnerability and trust that not everyone's past has afforded them? Do we know the differences between psychological dissociation from emotional overwhelm, and "checking out" from physical pain? Helping social workers better understand what questions to ask (e.g., *What have you been through and how has it impacted you?* vs. *What is wrong with you?*) can elevate the level of clinical intervention provided to our most vulnerable patients. There is a distinct chapter introducing the paradigm shift to this approach, but we have also attempted to integrate it throughout each individual chapter's approach to specific illness.

We hope this book provides an opportunity for critical reflection and clinical skill development for social workers in healthcare. We hope social workers recognize themselves and their skills in this book, see opportunities and directions for growth, and feel more empowered in how they understand their own roles and potential. This book shares practice wisdom, professional reflections, and an integration of literature and research that required the dedication, expertise, and novel thinking of two dozen social workers, to whom we give our deepest gratitude for their part in bringing this project to fruition.

New York, NY, USA

Meredith Hemphill
Abigail Nathanson

Acknowledgments

In appreciation of the wisdom, faith, patience and guidance of our mentors, Drs. Susan Gerbino and Carol Tosone.

In memory of health social work thought leaders and advocates, Zelda Foster and Helen Rehr.

With gratitude to the authors of the chapters in this book and to New York University Silver School of Social Work, where we met, learned and continue to grow.

For the students and social workers entering this field: a warm welcome! You have our heartfelt support, and we're glad you're here.

Contents

About the Editors

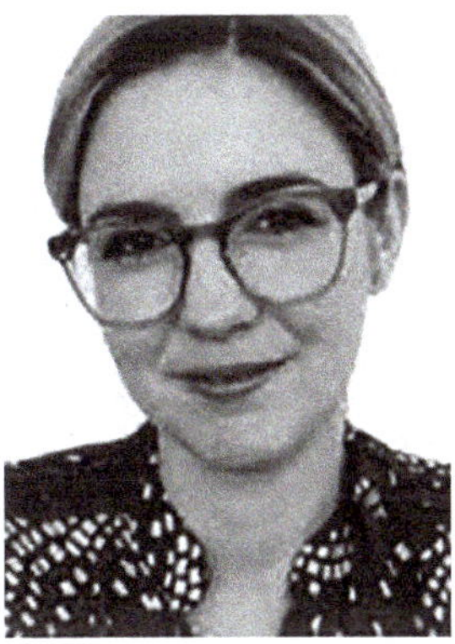

Meredith Hemphill, LCSW-R, DSW (she/her/hers), works as a Clinical Director and Director of Community Relations at City Center Psychotherapy in New York City. She teaches within the social work programs at New York University and Columbia University, and is a graduate of the Zelda Foster certificate program in Palliative and End-of-Life Care. She received her master's and doctoral degrees in social work from New York University, and bachelor's degree at Brown University. She has acted as a Guest Editor for the *Clinical Social Work Journal* for a special issue on social work in healthcare. Dr. Hemphill has contributed research and writing on the topic of hope-centered work with cancer patients, counseling during the COVID-19 pandemic and teaching grief and loss in social work education. She founded The Feather Foundation, a non-profit organization for parents who have cancer.

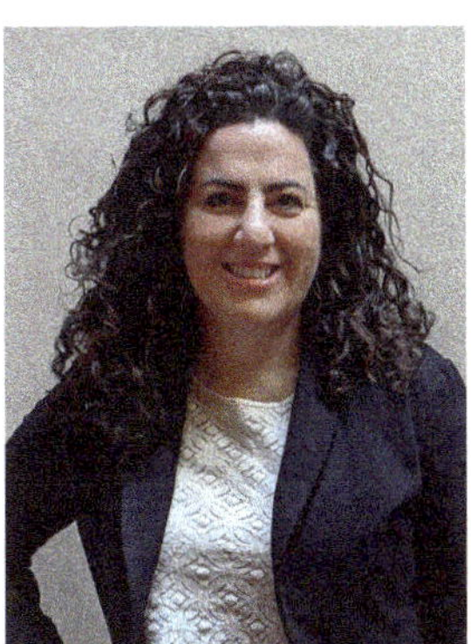

Abigail Nathanson, LCSW, DSW, APHSW-C, ACS (she/her/hers), is a palliative social worker and the founder of a trauma therapy practice specializing in illness, caregiving and loss. She is a part-time faculty member at New York University, where she teaches Grief, Loss and Bereavement, and a faculty member of the Zelda Foster Studies Program in Palliative and End-of-Life Care. She holds national board certification in palliative care, and has advanced training in Accelerated Experiential Dynamic Psychotherapy, EMDR and Meaning-Centered Psychotherapy. She worked in healthcare for 15 years, and has presented in grand rounds and division trainings in major academic medical centers across the country and published on topics relating to trauma, healthcare, bereavement, and death anxiety. Dr. Nathanson received both her master's and doctoral degrees in social work from New York University, and is the 2022 award recipient of the Social Work in Hospice and Palliative Network's Professional Educator of the Year.

Contributors

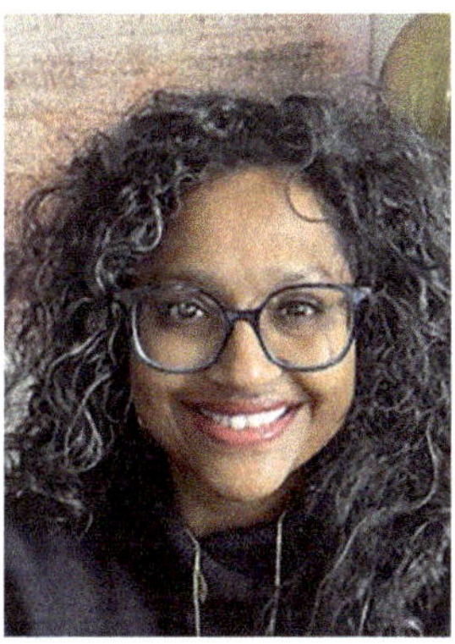

Annamma Abraham Kaba, LCSW-R is a manager and clinical supervisor, who oversees the Resources for Life After Cancer, a resource and counseling program for adult cancer survivors at Memorial Sloan Kettering Cancer Center. She has expertise in cancer survivorship, recognizing and supporting family caregivers and understanding how patients and families relate to their vulnerability and adversity during illness. Annamma has particular interest in psycho-spirituality and its role in the cancer experience. Annamma is a dedicated anti-racist practitioner and pursuing the development of anti-racist practices in healthcare. She graduated from Columbia University School of Social Work with a Master of Science and has a post-master's fellowship training in Gestalt Psychotherapy. Annamma joined Memorial Sloan Kettering in 1998 with extensive experience in both ambulatory and inpatient settings.

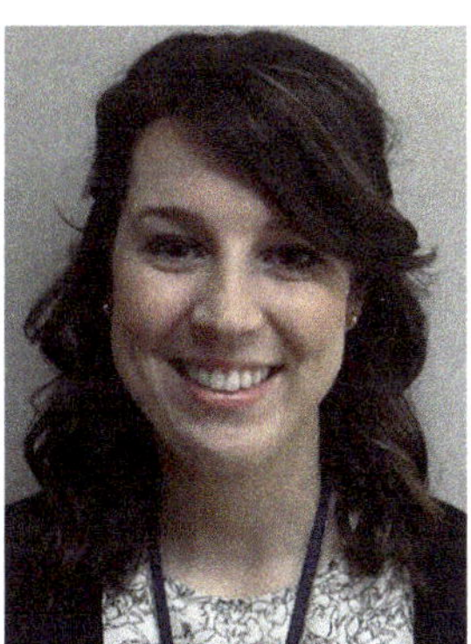

Chelsea K. Brown, LCSW, CCTP (Division of Palliative Medicine, University of California, San Francisco), is a licensed clinical social worker with the Inpatient Palliative Care Service at University of California, San Francisco (UCSF). She is also a current Leadership Fellow with the Zelda Foster Studies Program in Palliative and End-of-Life Care at New York University (NYU). Chelsea earned her master's degree from the University of Michigan School of Social Work after completing her clinical internship with the Inpatient Hematology Service. She has served in various social work capacities within and outside of the hospital setting, including: crisis and trauma intervention, community service connection, hospital social work, and now palliative care practice for patients and families living with serious illness.

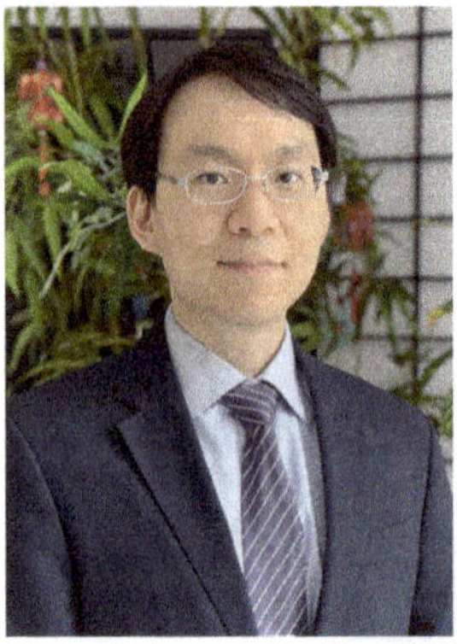

Peter (Tse Jen) Chu, LMSW is a social worker whose work focuses on taking care of patients with life-threatening illnesses. Prior to joining Coalition of Asian-American Independent Practice Associations (CAIPA), he was a senior reporter at *World* journal and won a 2018 Ippies Award for Best Investigative/In-depth Story. Witnessing the increased demand for mental health services in new immigrant communities, he made the career change to social work in 2018 and was selected for Palliative Care Fellowship at Fordham University, where he graduated with his MSW in 2020.

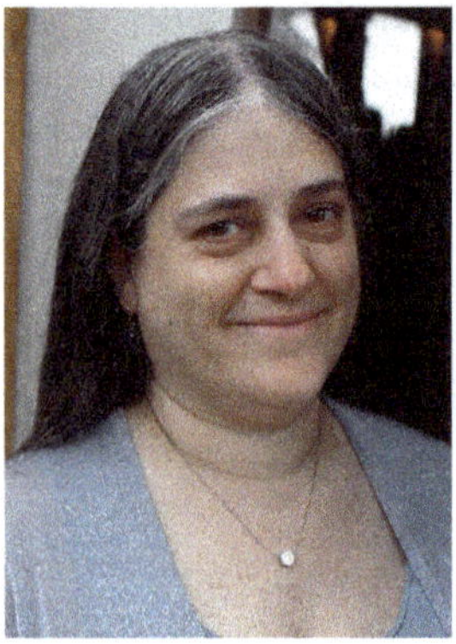

Nancy F. Cincotta, LCSW, MPhil, CLS is currently a Psychosocial Consultant in New York working with non-profit organizations and hospitals. Ms. Cincotta worked as a supervisor and clinician in the Division of Maternal Child Health at the Mount Sinai Medical Center for three decades and served as the Psychosocial Director at Camp Sunshine. She is a Senior Lecturer at the Columbia University School of Social Work, on faculty and a Mentor in the Zelda Foster Studies Program at New York University, and an Advisor in the Postgraduate Certificate Program in Palliative and End-of-Life Care, Smith College. She serves as a Clinical Consultant to the master's degree Genetic Counseling Program at Mount Sinai Health System, and is the Social Work Education and Research Coordinator at the Ovarian Cancer Research Alliance. Ms. Cincotta is a Past President of the Association of Pediatric Oncology Social Workers and has served as a Board Member with multiple professional and non-profit organizations. Ms. Cincotta received the Lifetime Contribution Award from the Association of Pediatric Oncology Social Workers (2016), The Inaugural Leukemia and Lymphoma Society Hematology/Oncology Lifetime Achievement Award, Association of Oncology Social Work (2019), and Outstanding Education and Training Award, American Psychosocial Oncology Society (2019).

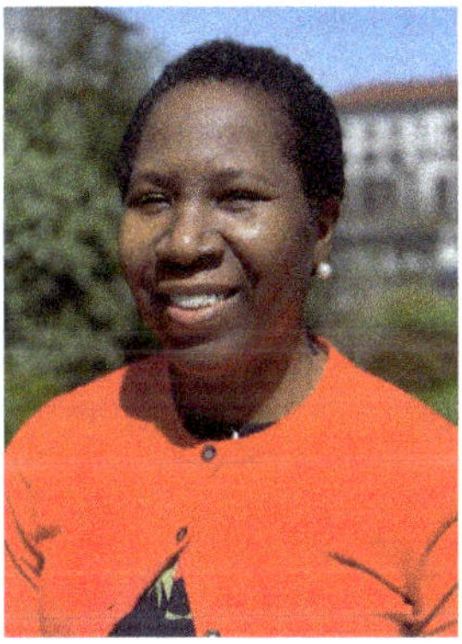

Marsha Clarke, LCSW is a licensed clinical social worker with over 21 years of direct care practice experience within healthcare. She has a master's degree from Hunter College Silberman School of Social Work. Her areas of expertise include Oncology, Palliative Care and Hospice, Home Care and Hospital discharge planning. She has completed leadership training through NYU Zelda Foster Studies Program in Palliative and End-of-life Care and served as a Zelda Foster Mentor. She is currently employed at Emory University Healthcare Hospital in the Cardiovascular Intensive Care Unit, providing clinical and discharge planning support to patients/families with complex surgical management and pre-transplantation, ECMO and LVAD needs. She also leads a case conference group for the Social Work Department. Marsha is a dedicated anti-racist clinician who is focused on facilitating the development of anti-racist practice within healthcare.

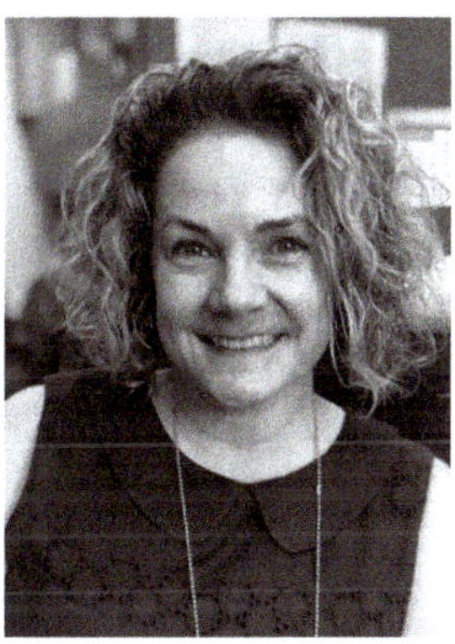

Diana M. Cory, MS Ed, MSW, LCSW (she/her/hers), is a licensed clinical social worker in the Division of Clinical Genetics, Department of Pediatrics, Columbia University Vagelos College of Physicians and Surgeons and previously worked at the Naomi Berrie Diabetes Center at Columbia University Irving Medical Center. She has master's degrees from Hunter College Silberman School of Social Work and from Bank Street Graduate School of Education. Ms. Cory is a member of the Diversity, Equity and Inclusion Working Group at National Organization for Rare Disorders (NORD). Ms. Cory's primary focus is to support her patients as they navigate new and rare genetic diagnoses, fostering meaningful connection between these patients and their families in order to best address their overwhelming social, emotional and often complex medical needs.

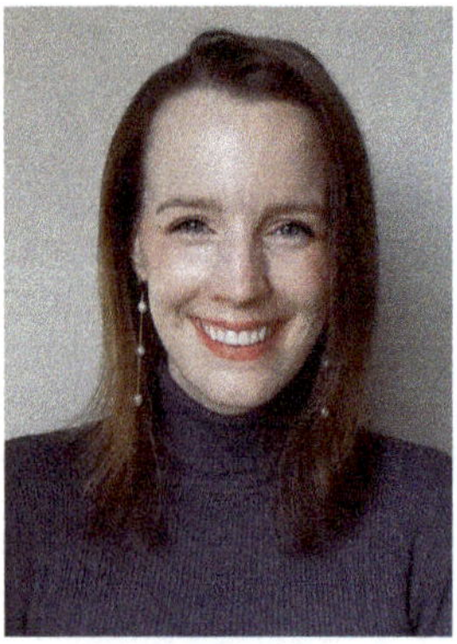

Jessica Desai, LCSW (she/her/hers), is a licensed clinical social worker currently working in private practice, focusing on areas including coping with illness, end-of-life and grief. Jessica received her master's degree from New York University and was an MSW fellow in the Zelda Foster Studies Program in Palliative and End-of-Life Care. Jessica's professional work has spanned hospital and community settings as an oncology and palliative care social worker.

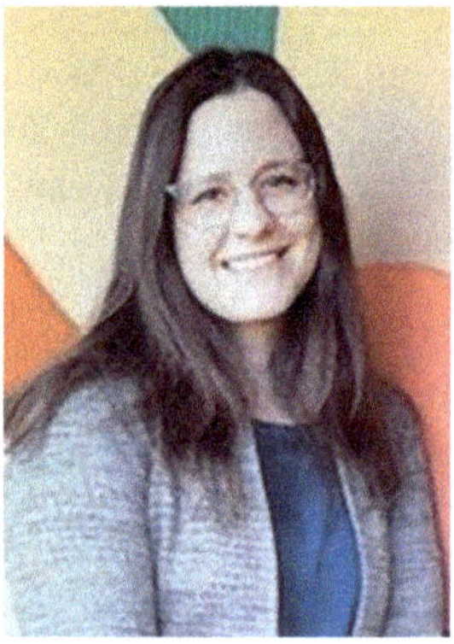

Jennifer DiBiase, LCSW-R, APHSW-C, DSW (she/her/hers), is a clinical social worker and manager for Mount Sinai Beth Israel's Department of Geriatrics and Palliative Care, providing care to patients in both the inpatient and outpatient settings and directing the post-master's palliative care social work fellowship. Throughout her career, she has focused her direct clinical practice, clinical supervision and coaching of interdisciplinary teams in support of patients and families coping with serious life-limiting illness. After nearly a decade working with Veterans and several years working with survivors of acute sexual assault, she understands how trauma impacts health behaviors, partnering with patients to help them navigate our complex medical system. She received her MSW at the University of California Berkeley in 2004 and received her doctorate in clinical social work at NYU in 2023.

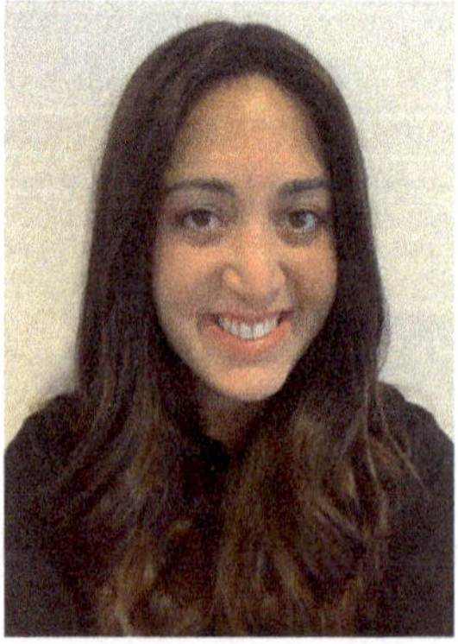

Maya Joyandeh, LMSW is a licensed social worker who received her master's degree from New York University in 2012. From 2011 to 2015, Maya was an MSW fellow in the Zelda Foster Studies Program in Palliative and End-of-Life Care at NYU and a JFEW Tannenbaum Fellow. For 10 years, she dedicated her practice to individuals receiving Hospice Care, as well as work within nursing homes, hospitals and homecare settings. Maya is now a Regional Field Director for Teach NJ, engaging the community and local nonpublic schools in the fight for government funding for education and school programs.

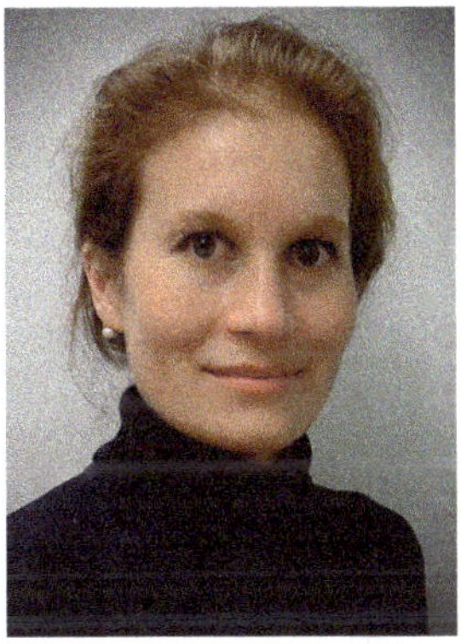

Zoe A. Landers, LCSW is a certified Sensorimotor Psychotherapy clinician and EMDR Consultant-in-Training. Zoe maintains a full-time private practice in New York City specializing in the treatment of complex posttraumatic stress, dissociation and eating disorders. Prior to developing a trauma-informed social work position at the Center for Brachial Plexus and Traumatic Nerve Injury at the Hospital for Special Surgery, Zoe worked with survivors of sexual assault, domestic violence, trafficking and war crimes at St. Luke's-Roosevelt Hospital, Safe Horizons and the Jewish Board of Family and Children Services. Postgraduate clinical training in the treatment of eating disorders and psychological trauma was completed through the Institute of Contemporary Psychotherapy, where Zoe also served a three-year term as the Co-Director of the Trauma Studies Center amongst other concurrent leadership roles.

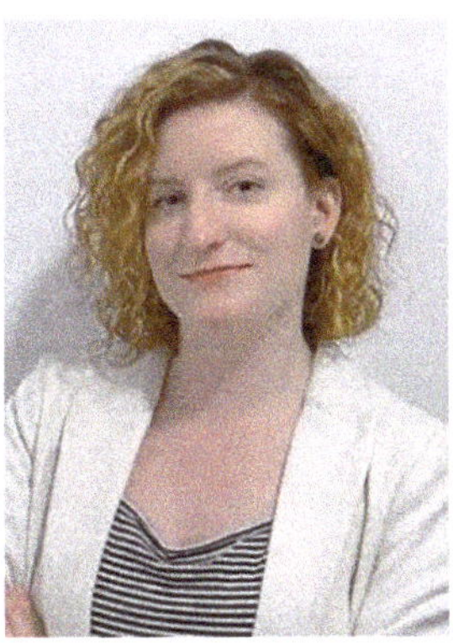

Sheila Langan, LMSW (she/her/hers), is a social worker with the Supportive Care Service at Memorial Sloan Kettering Cancer Center, where she works with oncology patients and the important people in their lives as they navigate serious illness. Prior to this, she worked with patients and caregivers facing dementia. A graduate of the NYU Silver School of Social Work and a former Zelda Foster MSW Fellow in Palliative and End-of-Life Care, Sheila completed a post-graduate fellowship in Palliative Social Work at Montefiore Medical Center and holds advanced certification in Bioethics and Medical Humanities.

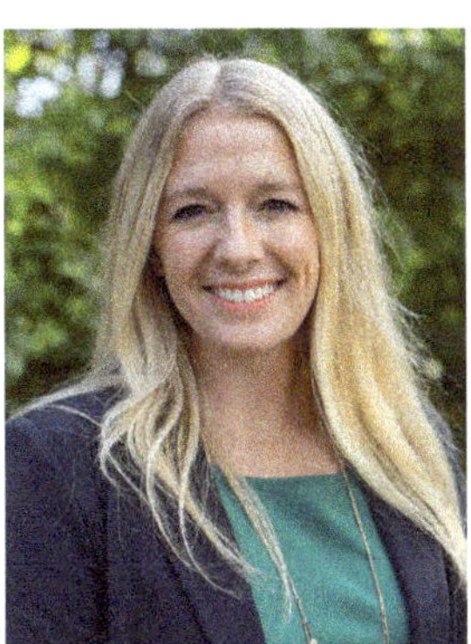

Abigail L. Latimer, LCSW, APHSW, PhD is an Assistant Professor in the College of Nursing with the University of Kentucky (UK) teaching in the MSN and DNP programs and jointly appointed at UK HealthCare as an Outpatient Palliative Clinical Social Worker. She received her BA in Psychology, is a Master of Social Work and Doctor of Philosophy in Social Work and completed post-doctoral training with the Research and Interventions for Cardiovascular Health (RICH) Heart Program at UK. Her clinical specialty is psychosocial and mental health care for patients with serious illnesses, and she has experience in behavioral health counseling for persons with addiction with over 7 years of experience in palliative and hospice care. Her research is centered on geriatric palliative care, with projects focused on serious illness communication, heart failure, older adults and clinicians' moral distress.

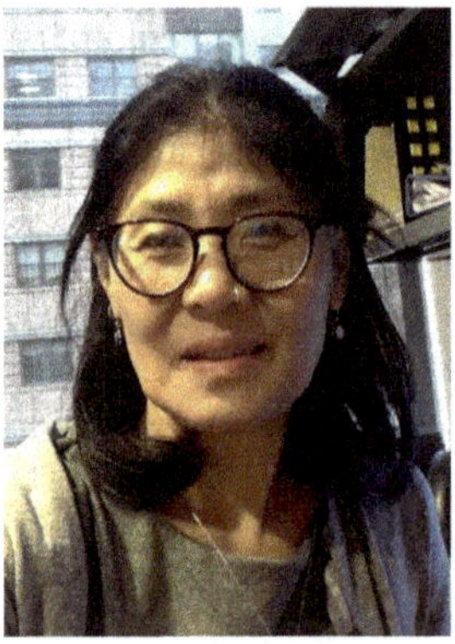

Eunju Lee, MSW, LCSW, MSOD, APHSW-C has worked in hospice and end-of-life care for the past 15 years. She is a mentor and faculty of NYU's Zelda Foster's Palliative and End-of-Life program and teaches palliative care at Fordham's online MSW program. She is also a leadership trainer for the Educating Social Workers in Palliative and End-of-Life Care (ESPEC) training program and continues to do clinical work at Memorial Sloan Kettering Cancer Center. She serves on the board of the Social Work in Palliative and Hospice Network and on its Health Equity Committee, and sits on the Healthcare Advisory Council for Compassion and Choices.

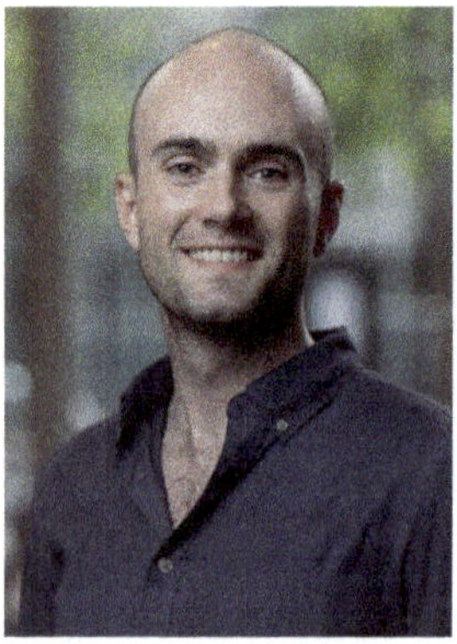

Jacob Maier, LCSW is a clinical social worker II at Memorial Sloan Kettering Cancer Center in the ambulatory outpatient setting. In addition, he has extensive experience working in the inpatient setting, specifically, on the Bone Marrow Transplant and Urgent Care Center services. Jake is also passionate about caregiver support and is co-leader of the Social Work Department's 'REACH for Caregivers' program which provides support groups, guided meditation sessions and other support opportunities to caregivers across all diagnoses. He completed his post-master's certificate in Palliative and End-of-Life care through NYU's Zelda Foster Leadership program. Jake received his master's degree in social work from NYU in 2018. Jake is a clinician who is dedicated to developing an antiracist practice within healthcare.

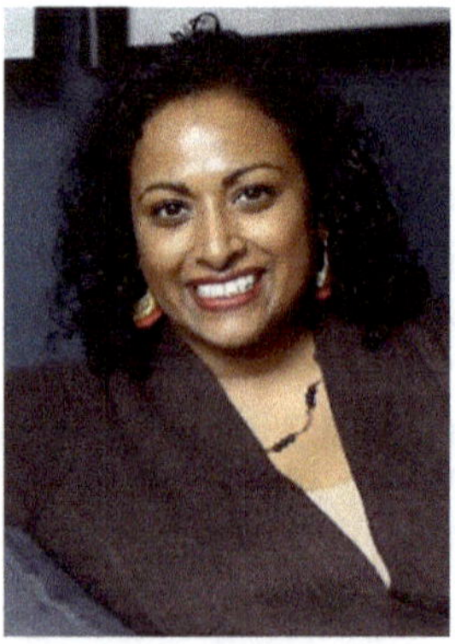

Linda Mathew, LCSW-R, DSW is a manager and clinical supervisor at Memorial Sloan Kettering Cancer Center. She earned her Master of Social Work degree in 2001 from New York University and completed her Doctor of Clinical Social Work degree at NYU in 2023. She is certified in Palliative and End-of-Life Care, Meaning Centered Psychotherapy, Cognitive Behavioral Therapy and Dialectic Behavioral Therapy. She has particular interest in supporting caregivers as well as children who have a parent diagnosed with cancer. She is a mentor and part-time faculty member of NYU's Zelda

Foster's Palliative and End-of-Life Program. Linda completed a three-year position on the Board of Directors for the Association of Oncology Social Workers as Director of Special Interest Groups. Linda is a clinician who is dedicated to developing an anti-racist practice within healthcare.

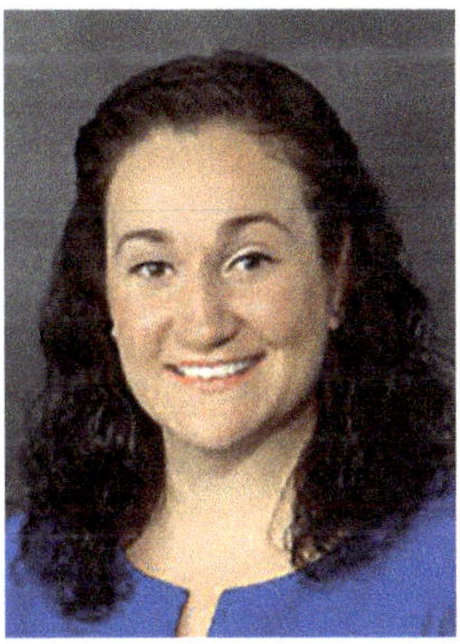

Caitlin Mayton, LCSW (she/her/hers), is a doctoral social work student at Virginia Commonwealth University (VCU) studying health inequities and the impact of historical trauma experienced by kidney transplant patients. Caitlin is actively working on two research teams, one based at Colorado University Anschutz Medical Campus focusing on inequities facing LVAD and heart transplant patients and social workers. The second is at VCU, where Caitlin participated in validating a curriculum (LEAP) on healthy relationships for people with disabilities. Previously, she earned her master's degree at the University of North Carolina at Chapel Hill School of Social Work. There she completed her clinical internship at Duke Medical Center with the heart transplant and LVAD service. After graduation, she worked at UNC Medical center in the transplant department as a licensed clinical social worker and certified transplant social worker for 5 years.

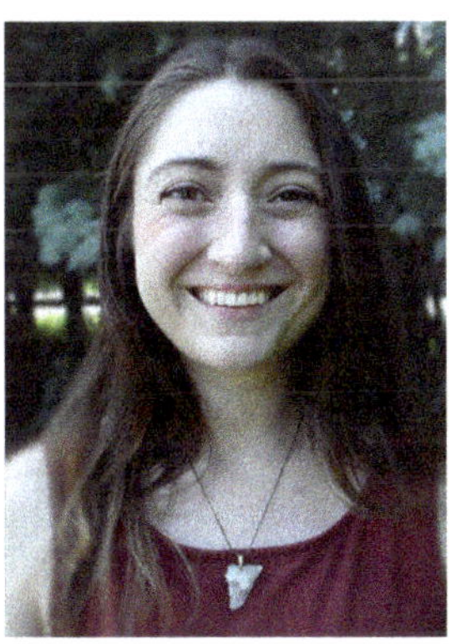

Kaila N. Robertson, MSW, LMSW is a social worker at Westchester Medical Center Advanced Physician Services where she supports patients in the post-COVID-19 Recovery Program. Prior to joining Westchester Medical Center, Kaila worked as an oncology social worker at Gilda's Club Westchester and as a therapist in a group practice. Kaila graduated from New York University Silver School of Social Work in 2021 where she was a fellow in the Zelda Foster Studies in Palliative and End-of-Life Care Program.

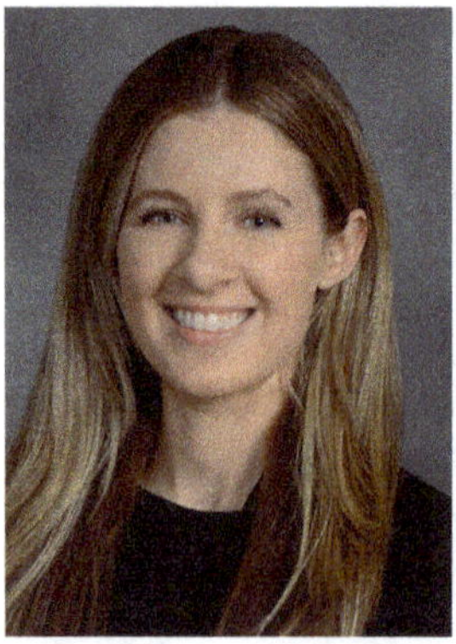

Madeline Rogers, MSW is a licensed social worker and interventionist with multifarious experiences in clinical research, direct clinical practice, training and case management, with a focus on bereavement, grief, palliative and end-of-life care. As a Research Program Coordinator-Interventionist at the New York Presbyterian-Weill Cornell Medicine Center for Research on End-of-Life Care, Ms. Rogers delivers therapeutic interventions on several nationally funded (NIMH, NIA, NCI, NINR) research studies and publishes widely on these topics.

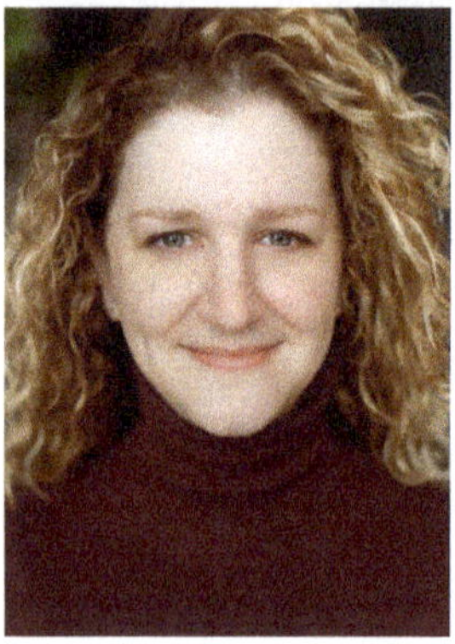

Rachel Rusch, MSW, LCSW, MA, APHSW-C (she/her/hers), is the Palliative Care Education and Practice Coordinator with the Division of Comfort and Palliative Care at Children's Hospital Los Angeles. Her career experience includes pediatric palliative care clinical social work and early childhood development. She is a recipient of the Cambia Health Foundation Sojourn's Scholar Leadership Program grant and a graduate of the Harvard Interprofessional Palliative Care Fellowship, specializing in pediatric palliative care. Named the 2020 Emerging Leader in Clinical Practice by the Social Work Hospice and Palliative Care Network, her research and program building initiatives center on the power of story, narrative and the humanities in health care.

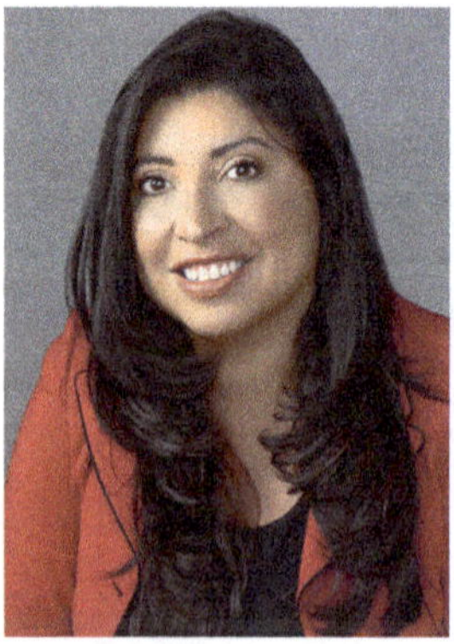

Erica Priscilla Sandoval, LCSW is a mental health practitioner, speaker, entrepreneur, philanthropist and author of *Latinx/e in Social Work* Volumes I and II, published in both English and Spanish. She served as Program Coordinator for the Department of Rheumatology at the Hospital for Special Surgery in New York City, and former President of the National Association of Social Workers, New York City chapter. Most recently, she is the founder and CEO of Sandoval Psychotherapy Consultation – known as Sandoval CoLab – where she oversees a team of social workers and leads diversity, equity and inclusion work for organizations, universities, healthcare facilities and medical and corporate professionals. Erica holds a post-master's in clinical adolescent psychology and a master's in social work from the New York University Silver School of Social Work. As a proud immigrant from Ecuador, her passion is fueled by supporting the community she is a part of and their children.

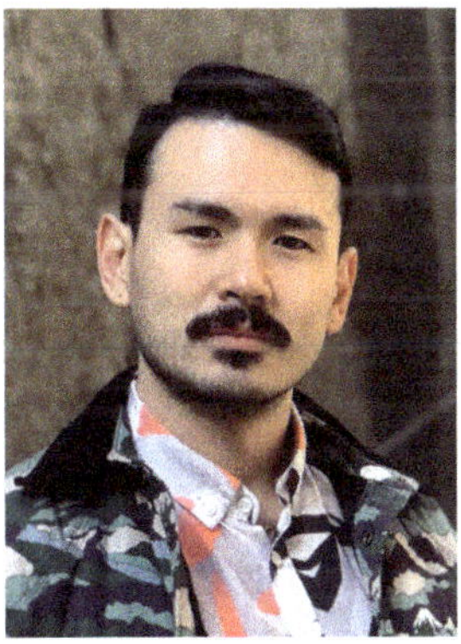

Andy Schlesinger, LMSW (he/him/his), is a psychotherapist at Callen-Lorde, an integrated community health center dedicated to serving the LGBTQ community in NYC. Previously, he was a social worker at the Manhattan VA Medical Center, where he worked in inpatient palliative care and with caregivers of veterans with serious illness and injury, and was a writer at the ACLU. He is a graduate of Columbia University and NYU Silver School of Social Work, where he was a fellow in the Zelda Foster Studies Program in End-of-Life and Palliative Care.

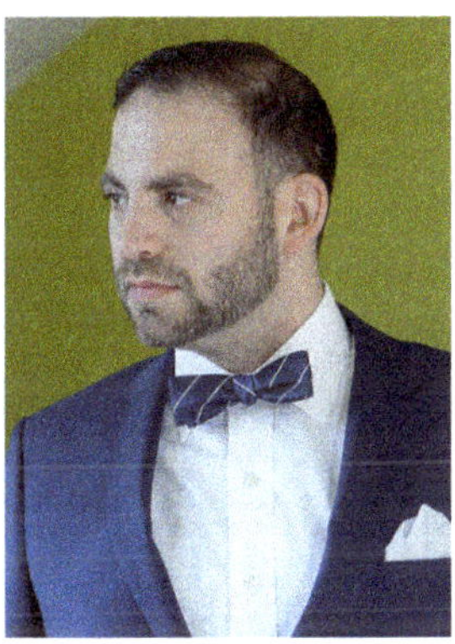

Adam Schoenfarber, LCSW, APHSW-C (he/him/his), is a palliative care and end of life social worker whose work focuses on narrative and existential techniques to help patients and families shape the stories they tell about themselves. He is currently the palliative care social worker at Westchester Medical Center in Valhalla and an Adjunct Lecturer at Fordham University. He has advanced training in Motivational Interviewing and Meaning-Centered Psychotherapy. He holds certifications in palliative care and Lean Six Sigma for Healthcare. He completed his master's at Columbia School of Social Work.

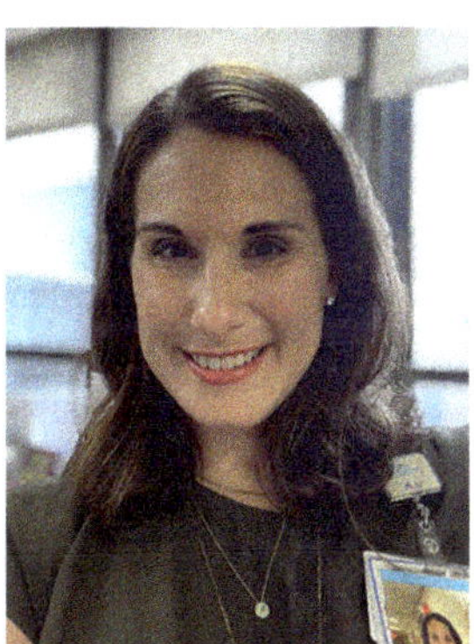

Alicia Tennenbaum, LCSW is the Executive Director of Social Work and Care Transitions at Mount Sinai Health at Mount Sinai Health System. Previously, she worked as Senior Director of the Department of Social Work and Case Management for the Mount Sinai Beth Israel, Mount Sinai Union Square and Mount Sinai New York Eye and Ear Campuses. She has served as a Date Rape/Domestic Violence victim advocate for the Beth Israel Victim Services Department and developed a prevention education program for schools on the topics of Date Rape and Healthy Relationship. She is currently a board member for the NYC chapter of the American Case Management Association. She was profiled in 2017 in the New York Times the gaps of care between hospital and home. She has co-authored a chapter on preparing for your discharge in 2008. She is a graduate of the Cornell-HANYS Academy for Healthcare Leadership Advancement (2014). She has her certificate in the field of Bioethics (2018) and is currently on the Ethics committee. She is a 2018 recipient of the Mount Sinai Heart Award and the Society for Social Work Leadership in Health Care, Ida M. Cannon Award, 2022.

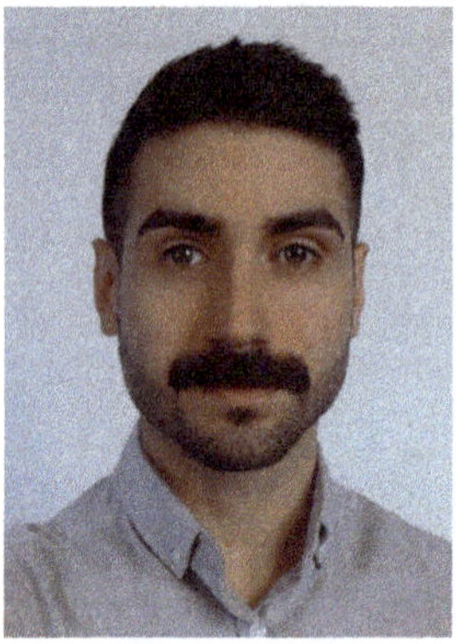

Richard Wenthen, LMSW (they/them/their), is a program manager with Community and Population Health at Northwell Health focusing on mental health and access to education with prior experience as a medical social worker at Lenox Hill Hospital specializing in neurosurgical and traumatic injury patient populations. Richard has a background as a professional performer and utilizes an embodiment perspective through a social justice lens with experience across the social work micro-macro spectrum. Richard holds a Master of Social Work from New York University and a Bachelor of Arts from Hofstra University.

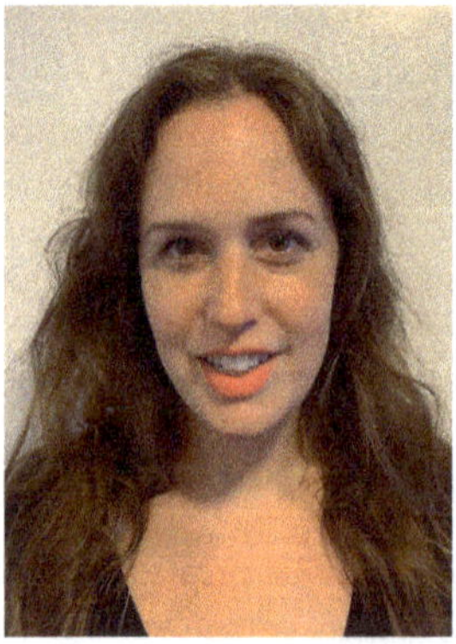

Michelle Willoughby, LCSW, DSW, ACM, ACSW (she/her/hers), is an Adjunct Instructor at New York University Silver School of Social Work. Michelle has more than a decade of experience as a social worker in NYC hospitals, coordinating support services for patients and families, and has received awards for her work. She has also supervised MSW interns and Columbia first-year medical students. Michelle earned her doctorate in social welfare at New York University and has published about her efforts as a hospital social worker during the COVID-19 pandemic. Michelle's professional goals are currently focused on building more partnerships between social work and libraries and incorporating biophilia into social work practice.

Chapter 1
Autoimmune Diseases

Jessica Desai and Erica Priscilla Sandoval

Introduction

Autoimmune diseases are illnesses affecting a person's immune system. More specifically, in patients with such illnesses, the immune system mistakes the patient's own tissue for a harmful invader such as a virus or bacteria, causing an immune response attacking healthy cells (MedlinePlus, 2021; National Institute of Arthritis and Musculoskeletal and Skin Diseases [NIAMS], 2016; National Institute of Environmental Health Sciences (NIEHS), 2021; Office on Women's Health, 2019). This process can affect several different areas of the body, depending on the type of autoimmune disease the person is diagnosed with. Four commonly known autoimmune diseases are rheumatoid arthritis (RA), lupus, multiple sclerosis (MS), and fibromyalgia. However, there are more than 80 known types of autoimmune disease affecting over 23.5 million Americans, predominantly women and those of African American, Hispanic American, and Native American descent (MedlinePlus, 2021; Office on Women's Health, 2019). Although anyone at any age can be diagnosed with an autoimmune disease, some factors can increase risk. For instance, those with a family history of a certain disease, especially lupus and MS, are more likely to contract the illness themselves (Office on Women's Health, 2019). In addition, with diagnoses such as RA, likelihood of onset increases with age (Chandrashekara, 2014). There are also environmental factors and social determinants of health

J. Desai (✉)
Norwalk, CT, USA
e-mail: jessica@jessicadesai.com

E. P. Sandoval
Sandoval Psychotherapy Consultation, Astoria, NY, USA
e-mail: erica@sandovalcolab.com

M. Hemphill, A. Nathanson (eds.), *The Practice of Clinical Social Work in Healthcare*, Essential Clinical Social Work Series,
https://doi.org/10.1007/978-3-031-31650-0_1

(SDOH) that can increase the likelihood of getting an autoimmune disease, which will be discussed later in this chapter.

A universal theme of the onset of autoimmune diseases is difficulty of early detection and diagnosis. There are several overlapping symptoms, including inflammation, chronic pain, swelling, fatigue, muscle aches, and low fever. Because these symptoms can be caused by other diagnoses and many autoimmune disorders do not have specific markers, diagnosis is often a lengthy process for providers (Chandrashekara, 2014). This can complicate the course of the illness, as early intervention is a key factor for more beneficial health outcomes. For the patient, diagnostic delays can cause significant distress, as they may be experiencing feelings of defeat or helplessness due to having symptoms without a known cause. If a patient sees treatment as delayed, they may also feel frustration and be preoccupied with "what-if" questions about what could have been done to help in the time it took to figure out the correct diagnosis. This presents a unique opportunity for the social worker in the clinic or hospital setting to provide support around these feelings of distress. The social worker has the ability to play a key role during the onset of an autoimmune disease by providing support to the individual around navigating the uncertainty of diagnosis. The social worker can also advocate for the patient to ensure better access to specialist appointments or second opinions; the social worker can also hold space for the patient's frustration and other feelings that may arise. These are all aspects of the social work role during this phase. Holding space communicates to the patient that the patient has the right to have those feelings; acknowledging the presence of those feelings; and allowing them to be there normalizes them in the patient's perception.

The course of autoimmune diseases can be unpredictable and vary widely from person to person. Symptoms tend to cycle through episodic flares into periods of remission. For someone diagnosed with lupus, flares could happen frequently or years apart, and the seriousness can range from mild to debilitating (Centers for Disease Control and Prevention [CDC], 2018). Similarly, many of those diagnosed with MS are mildly affected; however, some can lose the ability to write, speak, or walk (National Institute of Neurological Disorders and Stroke [NINDS], 2019). This sense of uncertainty of progression and prognosis can contribute to a great deal of anxiety and helplessness for the patient. Social work interventions of holding space and providing emotional support for facing the unknown can contribute to positive coping for those facing these illnesses. It can also be helpful for the social worker to guide the patient in identifying things that are within their control as a way to empower them and help them regain a sense of autonomy over their lives.

The speed and likelihood of progression of autoimmune diseases vary based on factors such as the type of illness and whether early intervention has occurred. For instance, RA is often chronic with a slow progression into systemic disease, with the characteristic joint damage and subsequent functional decline typically occurring over a period of several years (Chandrashekara, 2014; Hazes, 2003; Scott et al., 2010). However, evidence for the majority of autoimmune illnesses indicates that early diagnosis and effective treatment will reduce progression and may result in lasting remission (CDC, 2018; Chandrashekara, 2014; NINDS, 2019). Most autoimmune diseases are considered to be chronic, meaning that they have no cure and treatment is focused on symptom management, delaying progression, and moving toward remission. Definitions of remission may vary, but for diseases such as RA, this may include no active joint inflammation, erosive or functional deterioration, reduced disease activity or pain, and preservation of the ability to engage in activities of daily living (Scott et al., 2010). Although RA and most other autoimmune diseases themselves are not considered to be terminal, clients living with these diseases tend to have higher mortality rates than the general population due to complications or progression affecting vital organs. Comorbidities play an important role in outcomes, as having a diagnosis of an autoimmune disease can complicate or hasten other diseases (Young et al., 2007). For example, uncontrolled active RA can cause cardiovascular diseases that can be life-threatening (Scott et al., 2010). Lupus, another autoimmune disease that itself is rarely terminal, can sometimes increase the risk for end-stage renal disease (ESRD), which can be terminal (Faurschou et al., 2006).

The degree of incapacitation varies for each person and is dependent upon the course of the disease. Chronic pain, stiffness, and fatigue are some of the most common symptoms of autoimmune disease that contribute to incapacitation. The specific part of the body affected may also influence the extent to which the disease is disabling. For instance, if the joints in the fingers are primarily affected, activities such as writing, typing, cooking, engaging in certain hobbies, or other tasks that require fine motor skills will become increasingly difficult. As other areas of the body are affected, mobility becomes more complicated and thus life for the individual becomes further limited. More progressive manifestations may cause weight loss, loss of muscle mass, and immune responses affecting other organs.

Patients may experience distress when encountering the threat of progression or even mortality from potential complications. Here, the social work role can include holding space for the client to process these fears. The medical social worker can also empower clients to regain a sense of control by formulating questions for their provider and partnering with the interdisciplinary team to establish a care plan that may help ward off progression.

Clinical Issues of Illness

The following section provides an overview of clinical issues that the medical social worker may come across when working with clients facing an autoimmune disease. A significant experience that individuals and their family and friends may encounter is a sense of loss. Whether grief lies in the anticipation of future disability or death or relates to current losses (e.g., loss of a previous sense of self, loss of functioning, and loss of an imagined future), understanding the impact of losses throughout the trajectory of the illnesses is crucial for social workers. Grief and loss will be addressed in further detail in the bereavement section of this chapter.

Crisis

Intrapersonal In the crisis period of pre-diagnosis through the early stages of the diagnostic phase, the patient may experience feelings of uncertainty, fear, and frustration. As highlighted earlier in the chapter, autoimmune diseases are characteristically difficult to diagnose, so there can be an extended period wherein the individual is facing an influx of symptoms with no clear cause. This can be incredibly frustrating for the client and may create feelings of helplessness; when there is a history of disenfranchisement and helplessness within the medical system due to gender, ethnic, or other identities, this feeling can be exceptionally triggering. Once diagnosed, there can also be feelings of fear and uncertainty for the future. Due to the unpredictable nature and fluctuation of symptom flares with autoimmune illnesses like MS and lupus, it can be common for the individual to have fears of losing their functionality (Cowan et al., 2020).

There exists a strong relationship between the mental health of the individual and the onset of autoimmune diseases. High levels of distress and/or a history of trauma can predispose an individual to a diagnosis of an autoimmune illness like fibromyalgia (Galvez-Sánchez et al., 2019). Additionally, as we know from earlier in the chapter, symptoms of autoimmune diseases tend to present in flares. Research demonstrates that not only can these flares cause emotional distress, but also that emotional distress can cause the onset of a flare (Dissanayake & Bertouch, 2010; Bode & Taal, 2015; Galvez-Sánchez et al., 2019). This can lead to a cycle of physical symptoms triggering emotional distress and begetting more physical symptoms. This scenario can feel overwhelming and inescapable to the individual, especially during the crisis phase when everything is new and they may have yet to learn ways to cope.

Interpersonal Those who are diagnosed with an autoimmune disease may appear healthy from the outside, especially at the early stages of the illness. Common symptoms including fatigue and pain may not be immediately obvious to those in the individual's environment, and therefore, these illnesses are often referred to as "invisible." This invisibility can lead to failure on the part of friends, family, and even healthcare providers to validate the patient's experience, as these outside observers may underestimate the severity of symptoms while the patient is suffering significantly (Singh & Hamid, 2021). Singh and Hamid's (2021) study on patients with fibromyalgia found that negative social responses including lack of understanding, criticism, or giving unhelpful advice can lead to adverse effects on mental and physical well-being (Singh & Hamid, 2021). Continued negative feedback from the external world can be detrimental to an individual's quality of life, as it can be increasingly difficult for them to get the social and emotional support needed to cope with the side effects of these illnesses.

At the onset/crisis stage, the patient's family and friends may share in their feelings of fear of the unknown. They may want to provide support but be unsure how, or feel anxious about potential role changes. For instance, when an individual first begins to have pain flare-ups from their rheumatoid arthritis, others in the household may need to take on more chores or other responsibilities. For individuals who live alone, figuring out other ways to get instrumental activities of daily living (IADL) needs met can be stressful. Fatigue from RA, lupus, MS, or fibromyalgia may limit one's ability to engage in their typical social roles. Partners, children, elderly parents, or roommates may begin to become caregivers. These role shifts can cause disequilibrium in the family or other close social systems. Uncertainty for the future can permeate to family and friends, as they may wonder how long these changes will last or if the disease will progress. In response, the patient can be acutely aware of these changes in social dynamics, potentially causing them to feel that they are a burden or strain on the family, if there is an available and assistive family network.

Cynthia, a 36-year-old Latinx cisgender woman, has been experiencing waves of widespread chronic pain and fatigue over the past several months. Cynthia lives with her partner Victoria and their 2-year-old daughter Lucia, working full time as a nurse and also enrolled in graduate school. Cynthia was referred to the social worker in her primary care physician's office for mental health support after meeting with multiple providers without being able to find the underlying cause of her pain and fatigue. She shares that the onset of her symptoms occurred about one month into starting school and that her symptoms seem to spike in severity coinciding with her level of stress, usually due to work, school, or caring for her young daughter. She expresses feelings of guilt that her partner has had to take on more of the parenting responsibilities during symptom flares, which has caused some conflict in their relationship. Cynthia reports with frustration that, after several medical consultations with different specialists and inconclusive blood work, some family and friends and providers dismissed her concerns, saying that she was taking on too many responsibilities, and that her symptoms were likely a physical manifestation of stress. Cynthia identified that she felt unheard and helpless. With Cynthia's permission, the medical social worker continues with assessing Cynthia and learns Cynthia is a survivor of a sexual assault that occurred a few years ago and Cynthia decided to not report it due to feelings of shame. The social worker also learns she has not processed her traumatic incident or shared it with anyone, due to feelings of guilt. Cynthia describes being the first in her family to attend college and graduate and become a professional. Cynthia shared she migrated from Ecuador at the age of 14 and had difficulty managing the educational system alone and assimilating to her new environment. Though Cynthia works in a healthcare setting and is educated she describes being the only Latinx person in the classroom and also struggles with feelings of inadequacy. As she pursues her degree, her pain levels have increased. Cynthia speaks with an accent and presents as soft spoken and reserved when she is at her medical appointments. The social worker provided validation to Cynthia for her symptoms and experiences with trauma and seeking care and partnered with the primary care physician to advocate for a referral to a rheumatologist. The rheumatologist does a full medical workup and diagnoses Cynthia with fibromyalgia.

Systems of Care It is understood that early diagnosis and treatment are most effective in helping to achieve a higher quality of life for those with autoimmune diseases. Late diagnosis or misdiagnosis, along with limited access or poor adherence to treatments, is associated with a greater risk of complications and lower quality of life (CDC, 2018). Thus, as highlighted in the case of Cynthia, part of the role of the medical social worker is to advocate for access to high-quality care and promote effective coordination of care. Additionally, because diagnosis can be difficult and unclear initially, another intervention typical for the medical social worker is to ensure space is provided for the patient to communicate their symptoms and needs to their medical team. Unfortunately, some medical professionals may invalidate a patient's experience with autoimmune and rheumatological disorders due to the "invisibility" of the disease, as seen in Cynthia's case (Singh & Hamid, 2021). Further, because there is no clear standard for diagnosing illnesses such as fibromyalgia, which carry the possibility of several complex symptoms and may exist alongside other comorbidities, physicians or other medical professionals may misdiagnose the patient (Bidari et al., 2018). Many patients may give up or begin to question the veracity of their symptom experiences. This can lead to patients getting multiple opinions from different practitioners until they are properly diagnosed, which can, in turn, delay the start of effective treatment, further complicating the course of the illness. Thus, the social worker promoting effective communication and advocating for timely care is vital.

Early intervention in the areas of mental health and emotional support is also important. Cowan et al. (2020) found that with individuals who have MS, seeking out information on their condition may increase the patient's perceived capacity to deal with their illness (Cowan et al., 2020). This style of actively coping, by learning more about their diagnosis from reputable sources, may empower the patient to regain a sense of control in their medical care. The patient may feel less out of control if they know what to expect and what types of questions they should be asking their team. This presents a great opportunity for the medical social worker to partner with the patient and assess if they are in a mental space to take this active coping route. It is important to communicate with the patient how much information they are comfortable knowing before moving forward, so as not to overwhelm the individual or go against their wishes. In Cynthia's case, it may be helpful for the medical social worker to continue to meet with her on a regular basis early on in order to assess mental health needs and provide support where appropriate. Given Cynthia's trauma history, a trusting relationship with the social worker can be a necessary mechanism for addressing intrapersonal barriers to accessing care and addressing her concerns and mistrust of the medical system.

Another recommendation, by Jones et al. (2017), is for clinicians to consider the family system as a whole, understand its functioning, and provide family based interventions as a standard practice (Jones et al., 2017). As autoimmune diseases affect the social system in which the patient finds themselves, it may be best to communicate anticipated changes and address any concerns before they arise. Healthy communication around everyone's needs can help the couple, family, or chosen